Green Smoothie Recipes to Kick-Start Your Health and Healing

How to Detoxify Your Body and Start Healing Today.

By

Brooke Goldner, M.D.

Published by Express Results, LLC Austin, TX

Printed in the United States of America First Printing October 2013

Revised January 2014 Version 14.01

Revised February 2017

Important Legal Notice And Disclaimer

This publication is intended to provide educational information with regard to the subject matter covered.

The reader of this course assumes all responsibility for the use of these materials and information Brooke Goldner, M.D. and Express Results, LLC assume no responsibility or liability whatsoever on behalf of any purchaser or reader of these materials.

The methodology, training, products, mentoring, or other teaching does not guarantee success and the results may vary

The information in this book should not substitute for medical care by a licensed practitioner.

Please notify your doctor about any nutritional or alternative therapy you intend to use.

Green Smoothies for Health and Healing:

The most important part of my healing program for Lupus is consuming large amounts of nourishing green smoothies. Drink them frequently, keeping your body well-nourished and energetic, and in a constant state of healing.

These are some recipes from my kitchen. Feel free to change them up according to your taste. You may like it sweeter and want to add more fruit or dates, or you may want to add some fresh herbs.

You can also change up the greens depending on your tastes and what you have available, like kale, spinach, mustard greens chard, dandelion green romaine lettuce etc. Kale is the most nutrient-dense and should be a frequent player in the rotation. If you don't have (or like) all of the ingredients, make a substitution or simply leave it out.

Awesome Greens that you can BLEND!

Green Kale
Lacinato Kale (a.k.a. Dino Kale)
Beet Greens
Collard Greens
Dandelion Greens
Pea Greens
Rainbow Chard
Red Chard
Red Mustard Greens
Russian Kale
Spinach
Sweet Potato Greens
Swiss Chard
Turnip Greens
Kohlrabi Greens

Try as many different types of greens as you can, and pick some favorites! Try to have kale at least a few times a week, as well as others that you enjoy. The most important part of green smoothies is the fact that you *drink* them! Therefore it is vital that you enjoy the way they taste so you feel motivated to make them a part of your daily routine.

As you explore the different recipes in this book, I encourage you to try your own recipes out too. Make sure the main ingredient is fresh greens and then add your own fruits and vegetables to taste. If you mess up and the taste isn't quite what you like, I have found adding bananas and/or almond milk is a miracle fix for bitter smoothies. Also the stems of kale and other greens tend to be bitter, so I recommend you remove them and just use the leaves. Chard stems are an exception, they are sweet. If you still find the flavors of the greens to be too strong, try milder greens like spinach.

You might want to start out with sweeter smoothies as you adjust to the taste of the greens. You will likely find that with time you start enjoying the taste of the greens and can cut back on your fruits and add more greens, which is more ideal.

I often add chlorella and spirulina to my smoothies, super nutritious super foods, but they are not necessary if you don't have access to them.

Fresh versus Frozen?

The purpose of these green smoothies is to get you to consume far more greens than you normally would by making them into a delicious drink. Therefore we want to preserve the nutrients in the greens as much as possible. When it comes to greens, use fresh, raw ingredients whenever possible. Frozen foods lose a lot of their nutrients and are not as healthy and revitalizing.

Now the fruit is "the spoonful of sugar to make the medicine go down" to quote Mary Poppins, so I am not as concerned about whether the fruit is frozen or fresh since we are using fruit for flavor and not to add to the total nutrient density.

If you use frozen fruit then you don't need to add ice, but if you use fresh fruit you definitely need the ice to keep from cooking those greens.
Make sure your produce is fresh and completely ripe, and make sure you remove any brown spots before blending.

Does it need to be Organic?

While I always think it is better to use organic ingredients if you can, you can get healthy using traditional ingredients as well.

In fact, when I healed myself from Lupus, I couldn't afford organic produce so I used all traditionally grown vegetables, GMOs pesticides and all.

The benefits of organic ingredients is that they have no harmful chemicals, they are not gentically altered, and perhaps most importantly, they tend to have more vitamins and minerals because they are grown in better soil.

But if organic produce is outside of your budget, do the best you can and still eat your greens!

What liquids should I use?

Unless specified otherwise, add filtered water to the listed ingredients until you reach ¾ way to the top of the vegetables in the blender, add a few ice cubes and blend for 2 minutes or until fully liquefied. If you use fresh wheat grass, add at least a cup of ice and blend for 5 minutes to blend up the fibrous grass. These blend times are meant for the Vitamix blender. If you have a less powerful blender, you will need to blend longer, using more ice as you go, to make sure the drink is completely liquefied.

If you like a thinner consistency, use more water. For creamy smoothies add avocado and/or bananas.

You can also use nut milks or coconut water instead of filtered water if you prefer. Some store bought nut milks are sweetened with cane sugar, so try to find sugar free (or make your own). Do not add sugar to your smoothie or other foods; instead use fruits and dates to achieve sweetness.

Do I need a Vitamix Blender?

I highly recommend you get a high-powered blender, such as a Vitamix or a Blendtec. These blenders blend at up to 250 miles per hour. This breaks open the cell walls of the foods you are blending, effectively dumping the nutrients into the smoothie and giving you a powerful boost of energy and vitality that is unmatched by less powerful blenders. Slower blenders will break food up into smaller pieces, which will give you health benefit, but not the same level as with the more powerful blenders.

The recipes that follow are measured out to fill a Vitamix blender carafe. To adapt the recipes to another blender, or to make a smaller serving, simply measure out your ingredients so that your blender has 75% greens, and 25% fruit/other ingredients. This is the ratio that we have had the greatest success with in our patients and clients.

Can I make my Smoothies ahead of time and Store them?

Green smoothies can be stored in the refrigerator for up to 24 hours. When they are left out, they degrade quickly. I usually add ice to my travel jars in addition to packing them in a cold storage box with ice packs to ensure freshness on the go.

Green Smoothie

Recipes

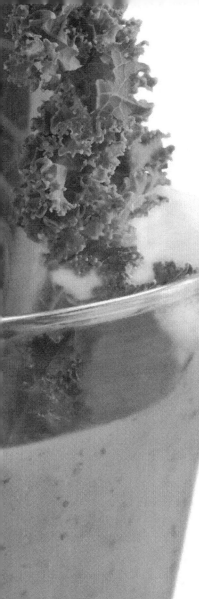

1. The Beginner

INGREDIENTS

This tasty smoothie makes a great first smoothie.

6 cups kale leaves,
1 pear
1 large banana,
1 cup of pineapple
1 avocado
Add almond milk 1/2 the way to the top of veggies
Optional 1 Handful flax seeds
Add water until 3/4 way to the top of the veggies.
Add 5 ice cubes

Doctor's orders

Blend for 2 minutes with a Vitamix until completely smooth, adding more ice halfway through blending to keep it cold.

If you have a less powerful blender, you will need to blend longer until it is completely blended, adding ice as needed to keep it cold.

2. Sweet Vanilla Banana Smoothie

A sweet delicious smoothie your kids (and you) will LOVE.

INGREDIENTS

1 banana
1/2 avocado
4 cups spinach
Optional 1 handful flax or chia seeds
Vanilla almond milk – fill 1/2 way to top of veggies. (If you don't have vanilla almond milk, you can use plain almond milk and add 1Tbsp of real vanilla extract)
Add water until ¾ from the top of veggies.
Add 5 ice cubes

Doctor's orders

Blend for 2 minutes with a Vitamix until completely smooth, adding more ice halfway through blending to keep it cold.

If you have a less powerful blender, you will need to blend longer until it is completely blended, adding ice as needed to keep it cold.

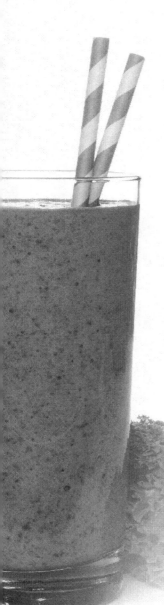

3. Rise and Shine Smoothie

Way better for you than orange juice and delicious all day long.

INGREDIENTS

5 tangerines (or 2 large oranges) peel removed
1 banana
2 carrots
6 cups green kale
Optional: 3000mg Chlorella
Optional: 1 handful flax seeds
Add water until ¾ from the top of veggies.
Add 5 ice cubes

Doctor's orders

Blend for 2 minutes with a Vitamix until completely smooth, adding more ice halfway through blending to keep it cold.

If you have a less powerful blender, you will need to blend longer until it is completely blended, adding ice as needed to keep it cold.

4. Beet me to the Green

Pears and beets give it a rich slightly sweet flavor.

INGREDIENTS

6 cups Black kale, stems removed
1 carrot
½ beet
1 celery stick
2 pears
Optional: 3000mg Chlorella
Optional: 1 handful flax seeds
Add water until ¾ from the top of veggies.
Add 5 ice cubes

Doctor's orders

Blend for 2 minutes with a Vitamix until completely smooth, adding more ice halfway through blending to keep it cold.

If you have a less powerful blender, you will need to blend longer until it is completely blended, adding ice as needed to keep it cold.

5. Fall for the Greens

This is an iron-rich smoothie with apples to add some delicious subtle sweetness.

INGREDIENTS

¼ cup fresh Parsley
5 cups Kale
2 carrots
2 red apples
Optional: 1 handful flax seeds
Add water until ¾ from the top of veggies.
Add 5 ice cubes

Doctor's orders

Blend for 2 minutes with a Vitamix until completely smooth, adding more ice halfway through blending to keep it cold.

If you have a less powerful blender, you will need to blend longer until it is completely blended, adding ice as needed to keep it cold.

6. Thomas's Simple Greens

Tart and smooth.

INGREDIENTS

2 granny smith apples
1 avocado
6 cups kale
Optional: 1 handful flax seeds
Add water until ¾ from the top of veggies.
Add 5 ice cubes

Doctor's orders

Blend for 2 minutes with a Vitamix until completely smooth, adding more ice halfway through blending to keep it cold.

If you have a less powerful blender, you will need to blend longer until it is completely blended, adding ice as needed to keep it cold.

7. Mean and Green

A savory treat with a garlic punch

INGREDIENTS

4 cups kale
2 cucumbers
2 celery stalks
1 avocado
3 Roma tomatoes
3 cloves garlic
Juice of 1 lemon or lime
Optional: 1 handful flax seeds
Add water until ¾ from the top of veggies.
Add 5 ice cubes

Doctor's orders

Blend for 2 minutes with a Vitamix until completely smooth, adding more ice halfway through blending to keep it cold.

If you have a less powerful blender, you will need to blend longer until it is completely blended, adding ice as needed to keep it cold.

8. Chocolate Dream Green

To satisfy your sweet tooth.
This is known by my son as "chocolate milk" in my house.

INGREDIENTS

¼ cup cacao powder
1 cup almond milk
1 cup filtered water
2 dates
1 avocado
4 cups collard green leaves
1 banana
Optional: 1 handful flax or chia seeds
Add 5 ice cubes

Doctor's orders

Blend for 2 minutes with a Vitamix until completely smooth, adding more ice halfway through blending to keep it cold.

If you have a less powerful blender, you will need to blend longer until it is completely blended, adding ice as needed to keep it cold.

9. Farmer's Market

Full of nutritious vegetables and greens for a savory smoothie.

INGREDIENTS

2 carrots
5 cups collard green leaves (or 6 small ones)
½ yellow squash
2 red apples
1 yellow pepper
½ avocado
½ of 1 beet.
Optional: 1 handful flax or chia seeds
Add water until ¾ from the top of veggies.
Add 5 ice cubes

Doctor's orders

Blend for 2 minutes with a Vitamix until completely smooth, adding more ice halfway through blending to keep it cold.

If you have a less powerful blender, you will need to blend longer until it is completely blended, adding ice as needed to keep it cold.

10. Refresh me

A great refreshing drink for a warm sunny day. Kids love them.

INGREDIENTS

2 ½ cups Watermelon
5 cups Green Kale
4 dates
Add water until ¾ from the top of veggies.
Add 5 ice cubes

Doctor's orders

Blend for 2 minutes with a Vitamix until completely smooth, adding more ice halfway through blending to keep it cold.

If you have a less powerful blender, you will need to blend longer until it is completely blended, adding ice as needed to keep it cold.

11. The Energizer

Drink this and feel energized and revitalized, POW!

INGREDIENTS

5 cups spinach
2 inch section of raw sweet potato with skin on
1 large avocado
½ cup fresh wheat grass
Optional: 2tbsp Spirulina
Optional: 1 handful Flax Seeds
Add water until ¾ from the top of veggies.
Add 5 ice cubes

Doctor's orders

Blend for 2 minutes with a Vitamix until completely smooth, adding more ice halfway through blending to keep it cold.

If you have a less powerful blender, you will need to blend longer until it is completely blended, adding ice as needed to keep it cold.

12. Super Green

Not looking for something sweet?
Try this one out.

INGREDIENTS

1 zucchini
3 Persian cucumbers,
1 avocado
4 cups spinach
4 mint leaves.
Optional: 1 handful Flax seeds
Optional: 3000mg Chlorella
Add water until ¾ from the top of veggies.
Add 5 ice cubes

Doctor's orders

Blend for 2 minutes with a Vitamix until completely smooth, adding more ice halfway through blending to keep it cold.

If you have a less powerful blender, you will need to blend longer until it is completely blended, adding ice as needed to keep it cold.

13. Greens Peas

For a mild tropical flavor.

INGREDIENTS

½ cup fresh peas
2 cups pineapple
5 cups red chard (stems removed)
2 baby bananas (or 1 regular banana)
Optional: 1 tsp Maca powder
Optional: 1 handful flax seeds
Add water until ¾ from the top of veggies.
Add 5 ice cubes

Doctor's orders

Blend for 2 minutes with a Vitamix until completely smooth, adding more ice halfway through blending to keep it cold.

If you have a less powerful blender, you will need to blend longer until it is completely blended, adding ice as needed to keep it cold.

14. Ginger Snap

I love the flavor of ginger!

INGREDIENTS

2 pears
1" section of ginger
6 cups kale
1 orange
Optional: 1 handful flax seeds
Add water until ¾ from the top of veggies.
Add 5 ice cubes

Doctor's orders

Blend for 2 minutes with a Vitamix until completely smooth, adding more ice halfway through blending to keep it cold.

If you have a less powerful blender, you will need to blend longer until it is completely blended, adding ice as needed to keep it cold.

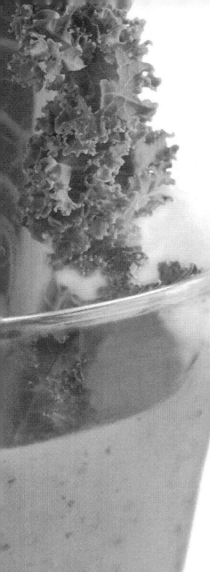

15. Green Energy

Wheat grass gives this smoothie an extra kick of energy!

INGREDIENTS

1 avocado
5 cups black kale
1/3 cup wheat grass
2 green apples
Optional: 1tbsp chlorella
Optional: 1 handful Flax seeds
Add water until ¾ from the top of veggies.
Add 5 ice cubes

Doctor's orders

Blend for 2 minutes with a Vitamix until completely smooth, adding more ice halfway through blending to keep it cold.

If you have a less powerful blender, you will need to blend longer until it is completely blended, adding ice as needed to keep it cold.

16. Green and Grape

Grapes add delicious sweetness.

INGREDIENTS

2 cups red grapes
1 whole banana
6 cups spinach
Optional: 1 handful flax seeds
Add water until ¾ from the top of veggies.
Add 5 ice cubes

Doctor's orders

Blend for 2 minutes with a Vitamix until completely smooth, adding more ice halfway through blending to keep it cold.

If you have a less powerful blender, you will need to blend longer until it is completely blended, adding ice as needed to keep it cold.

17. Orange you Grape

Mild sweetness without the bananas with a citrus zing.

INGREDIENTS

1 cup red grapes
1 orange
1 pear
2 stalks of celery
5 cups spinach
Optional: 1 handful flax seeds
Add water until ¾ from the top of veggies.
Add 5 ice cubes

Doctor's orders

Blend for 2 minutes with a Vitamix until completely smooth, adding more ice halfway through blending to keep it cold.

If you have a less powerful blender, you will need to blend longer until it is completely blended, adding ice as needed to keep it cold.

18. Apple-Strawberry Beet Greens

Strawberries, bananas and apples are a great mixture for a summertime smoothie.

INGREDIENTS

1 large apple
1 medium banana
1 cup whole strawberries (with greens)
6 cups beet greens
Optional: 1 handful flax or chia seeds
Add water until ¾ from the top of veggies.
Add 5 ice cubes

Doctor's orders

Blend for 2 minutes with a Vitamix until completely smooth, adding more ice halfway through blending to keep it cold.

If you have a less powerful blender, you will need to blend longer until it is completely blended, adding ice as needed to keep it cold.

19. Celery Smoothie

Celery adds a nice crisp flavor.

INGREDIENTS

5 cups spinach
2 green apples
3 mint leaves
3 celery stalks
Optional: ½ cup wheat grass
Optional: 1 handful flax seeds
Add water until ¾ from the top of veggies.
Add 5 ice cubes

Doctor's orders

Blend for 2 minutes with a Vitamix until completely smooth, adding more ice halfway through blending to keep it cold.

If you have a less powerful blender, you will need to blend longer until it is completely blended, adding ice as needed to keep it cold.

20. Orange you refreshed?

This is a favorite smoothie for a refreshing citrus flavor.

INGREDIENTS

6 tangerines, peeled
2 carrots (unpeeled)
Juice of 1 large lemon
1 avocado
5 cups black kale
Optional: 1 handful flax or chia seeds
Add water until ¾ from the top of veggies.
Add 5 ice cubes

Doctor's orders

Blend for 2 minutes with a Vitamix until completely smooth, adding more ice halfway through blending to keep it cold.

If you have a less powerful blender, you will need to blend longer until it is completely blended, adding ice as needed to keep it cold.

21. Blueberry Blast

Blueberries and apples give this smoothie an extra delicious punch of flavor!

INGREDIENTS

5 cups black kale
1 1/2 cup blueberries
2 sweet red apples
½ cup wheat grass
1 avocado
Optional: 1 handful flax or chia seeds
Optional: 300mg Chlorella
Add water until ¾ from the top of veggies.
Add 5 ice cubes

Doctor's orders

Blend for 2 minutes with a Vitamix until completely smooth, adding more ice halfway through blending to keep it cold.

If you have a less powerful blender, you will need to blend longer until it is completely blended, adding ice as needed to keep it cold.

22. Fruit delight

It's like a fruit bowl in a cup!

INGREDIENTS

6 cups kale
1 small green apple
2 bananas
1 pear
½ cup blueberries
Optional: 1 handful flax or chia seeds
Add water until ¾ from the top of veggies.
Add 5 ice cubes

Doctor's orders

Blend for 2 minutes with a Vitamix until completely smooth, adding more ice halfway through blending to keep it cold.

If you have a less powerful blender, you will need to blend longer until it is completely blended, adding ice as needed to keep it cold.

23. Green Zinger

Lettuce has a very mild taste, letting the fruit take the lead on your tastebuds!

INGREDIENTS

5 cups romaine lettuce
4 tangerines
1 pear
½ cup blueberries
Optional: ¼ cup wheat grass
Optional: 1 handful chia or flax seeds
Add water until ¾ from the top of veggies.
Add 5 ice cubes

Doctor's orders

Blend for 2 minutes with a Vitamix until completely smooth, adding more ice halfway through blending to keep it cold.

If you have a less powerful blender, you will need to blend longer until it is completely blended, adding ice as needed to keep it cold.

24. The Husband's Favorite

This is a great smoothie for anyone who likes a mix of sweet and tart. Also great for beginners, since the spinach is very mild and there is a lot of fruit.

INGREDIENTS

5 cups of spinach
2 green apples
1 cup of grapes
1 avocado
3 small bananas
Optional: 1 handful flax seeds
Add water until ¾ from the top of veggies.
Add 5 ice cubes

Doctor's orders

Blend for 2 minutes with a Vitamix until completely smooth, adding more ice halfway through blending to keep it cold.

If you have a less powerful blender, you will need to blend longer until it is completely blended, adding ice as needed to keep it cold.

Thank you for purchasing this book. I hope it brings you great health and delicious drinks!

While these green smoothies can drastically improve your health, you may still have residual disease, have difficulty healing fully, or have less than optimal energy levels if your diet contains foods that cause disease, or you are missing other vital healing foods.

I encourage you to continue your journey towards optimum health by continuing to learn as much as you can and be open to changing your habits and conquering food addictions.

My Best Selling book, Goodbye Lupus, contains the full story of how I reversed my disease, Lupus, and a simple step-by-step guide of how to eat to reverse inflammation and disease and optimize health.

If you would my help in taking back your health, I would love to be your guide. Feel free to email me any time, or you can go to my website for a consultation.

http://www.VeganMedicalDoctor.com

I wish you amazing fitness and health,

Brooke Goldner, M.D.

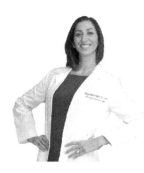

Made in United States
Troutdale, OR
10/24/2023

13957708R00022